Maximize Your Metabolism

Precision Nutrition and Fitness Techniques

Table of Contents

Chapter 1. Introduction

In the whirlwind world of wellness, there's an art and science to stoking the glorious furnace that is your metabolism. Our Special Report: "Maximize Your Metabolism: Precision Nutrition and Fitness Techniques" will empower you with knowledge and strategies to rev your metabolic engine to its optimum level. The report combines the latest research in nutrition and exercise science, and breaks it down into easy-to-understand strategies, enabling you to not only understand but practically use this precious information. Replete with expert tips and a wealth of scientifically-backed advice, this report will inspire you to unlock your body's full potential. Say goodbye to fad diets, and hello to sustainable health! Embark on this journey as we guide you to a healthier, energy-filled version of yourself. Who knew making peace with your metabolism could be so delightful! Purchase this Special Report today and watch yourself transform!

Chapter 2. Understanding Your Metabolic Machine

The intriguing machinery that is human metabolism plays an unsung but critical role in your overall health and well-being. Understanding this intricate process will provide glimpses into the dynamics of energy production and utilization in your body, explaining why certain nutrition and fitness techniques work while others don't.

2.1. The Basics of Metabolism

At its simplest, metabolism refers to the myriad chemical processes that occur within a living organism to maintain life. These processes enable our bodies to sustain life by doing jobs like converting food into energy for cells and waste materials to be disposed of. Metabolism is a complex system that comprises two main components: catabolism and anabolism.

Catabolism is the process of breaking down complex substances into simpler ones, releasing energy. It involves digestive enzymes that break down proteins in food into amino acids, fats into fatty acids, and carbohydrates into simple sugars like glucose. These broken components are then absorbed into the bloodstream, transported to cells, and broken down even further through cellular respiration, giving rise to energy.

Anabolism, on the other hand, is the process of building up or synthesizing complex substances from simpler ones. It involves the cells using the energy released by catabolism to construct components of cells such as proteins and nucleic acids.

2.2. Decoding Energy Balance

The continuous dance between catabolism and anabolism eventually determines your energy balance – the balance between the calories your body takes in and burns off. If you consume more calories than you burn, that extra energy gets stored, primarily as fat. Conversely, if you burn more calories than you consume, your body must draw on its energy stores, resulting in weight loss.

2.3. The Role of Basal Metabolic Rate

Integral to this understanding is the Basal Metabolic Rate (BMR), the number of calories your body needs to perform its most basic (basal) functions, such as breathing, circulation, cell production, nutrient processing, protein synthesis, and ion transport. Typically, your BMR accounts for around 60 to 75 percent of the total calories you burn each day.

Factors affecting BMR include age, sex, genetics, body composition (more muscle increases BMR), body size, and hormonal health. Understanding these factors can provide key insights into your metabolic health and aid in crafting personalized wellness strategies.

2.4. The Thermic Effect of Food

Another important concept in our metabolic discourse is the Thermic Effect of Food (TEF), which refers to the energy expended to digest, absorb, and distribute nutrients. Surprisingly, different macronutrients have different thermic effects. For instance, protein has a high thermic effect, meaning you burn more calories to digest proteins than carbohydrates or fats.

2.5. Physical Activity: The Movable Piece of The Puzzle

While BMR and TEF are relatively fixed, physical activity is the variable you can most easily manipulate to influence your energy expenditure. Any bodily movement—as easy as standing, walking to work, or as intensive as weight-lifting—burns calories, contributing to increased energy output. The type, duration, and intensity of exercise significantly influence this piece of your metabolic puzzle.

2.6. Hormones and Metabolism

Our endocrine system plays a significant role in metabolic regulations. Hormones such as insulin, glucagon, leptin, and ghrelin, among others, influence our appetite, satiety, how we metabolize different nutrients, and how we store energy. Disorders in these hormones can lead to metabolic imbalances and weight issues, highlighting the importance of hormonal health in metabolic wellness.

2.7. The Impact of Age and Sleep on Metabolism

As we age, our metabolic rate tends to slow down due to a decrease in muscle mass and increase in fat mass. This emphasizes the importance of resistance training to maintain or increase muscle mass with aging. Sleep also prominently impacts our metabolism. Lack of sleep or poor-quality sleep can disrupt our hormonal balance, further impacting our metabolic health.

2.8. The Metabolic Power of Hydration

Water plays a central role in every aspect of metabolism. It helps transport nutrients, hormones, and oxygen, facilitates the excretion of waste products, and maintains normal body temperature. Dehydration, therefore, could lead to a temporary metabolism slowdown.

2.9. Metabolism and Weight Loss

While we often blame a 'slow metabolism' for weight gain, research suggests it's rarely the primary cause of excess weight. Most weight gain occurs as a combination of genetic, hormonal, and environmental factors, along with lifestyle choices relating to diet and physical activity.

By understanding the intricate processes involved in metabolism and the factors that influence it, you're better equipped to optimize your metabolic health. Remember, the path to sustainable health and wellness is not through quick fixes or fad diets, but through understanding and embracing the complex machinery of your body, your metabolic machine.

Chapter 3. The Role of Precision Nutrition in Metabolism

Nutrition is one of the most vital factors that affect your metabolic rate, and precision nutrition, which caters to your unique nutritional needs based on individual characteristics such as genetics, lifestyle, and physical activity, can greatly enhance your metabolic efficiency. By understanding the role of precision nutrition in boosting metabolism, you can optimize your diet to suit your body's specific requirements, enabling you to burn calories more effectively.

3.1. Understanding Metabolism

Metabolism is a complex web of biochemical reactions essentially consisting of two main processes: anabolism (building up) and catabolism (breaking down). While the anabolic process utilizes energy to construct components of cells such as proteins and nucleic acids, the catabolic process breaks down organic matter to harvest energy in cellular respiration.

Your metabolic rate determines the amount of calories you burn in a day and is influenced by several factors. Basal Metabolic Rate (BMR) accounts for about 60-70% of total energy expenditure, largely determined by your age, gender, weight, and muscle mass. The rest is influenced by the thermic effect of food (TEF), physical activity, and other factors.

3.2. Precision Nutrition: A Tailored Approach

Precision nutrition is the concept of tailoring dietary recommendations to each individual's unique genetic, physiological, and lifestyle factors. This approach recognizes that every person's body responds differently to various types of foods and nutrients; hence, a "one-size-fits-all" diet plan may not be optimal for everyone. Precision nutrition aims to provide individuals with personalized nutrition advice rather than generalized dietary guidelines.

3.3. Macro and Micro: The Power of Nutrients

Macronutrients (carbohydrates, proteins, and fats) and micronutrients (vitamins and minerals) play vital roles in metabolic processes. Carbohydrates are the body's primary fuel and are essential for maintaining an optimal metabolic rate. Proteins are crucial for building and repairing body tissues, and they also have a thermogenic effect, meaning they can boost metabolism by raising your body temperature. Fats, especially omega-3 fatty acids, can optimize metabolic health by reducing inflammation and improving cellular function.

Micronutrients, though needed in smaller amounts, are equally vital. These include various vitamins, minerals and bioactive compounds, many of which can influence metabolism. For instance, B vitamins can help cellular metabolism by assisting in the breakdown of carbohydrates, proteins, and fats for energy. Minerals like iodine and selenium are essential for proper thyroid function, a gland that plays a crucial role in regulating metabolism.

In precision nutrition, knowing your unique nutritional needs, including the specific amounts, ratios, and types of these macronutrients and micronutrients that best suit your body, can help optimize your metabolism.

3.4. Tailored Meal Timing

Contrary to popular belief, when you eat can be just as important as what you eat. With precision nutrition, eating patterns can be strategized to align with the body's natural circadian rhythm, which can enhance metabolic efficiency. For instance, intermittent fasting, a dietary pattern that cycles between periods of eating and fasting, can help improve metabolic health by aligning eating schedules with your body's internal clock.

3.5. Genetic Influence: Your DNA Diet

Your genes can significantly influence the way you metabolize certain nutrients, which can affect your body weight, hunger levels, and overall health. Certain genetic variants can affect how your body responds to certain types of diets. For example, some people may metabolize fats more efficiently than carbohydrates, influencing which diet may result in weight loss for them. In precision nutrition, DNA testing can be used to design a personalized diet plan that capitalizes on your genetic strengths.

[[insert table]] .Table: Interaction of Genes and Diet

Gene	Effect	Dietary Advice
FTO	Increased appetite, preference for fat	Reduced calorie intake, higher protein diet
MC4R	Increased appetite, preference for fat	Reduced calorie intake

Gene	Effect	Dietary Advice
APOA5	Increased triglycerides	Reduced saturated and trans fat intake
LIPC	Increased HDL cholesterol	Increased monounsaturated fat intake

[[end of table]]

Precision nutrition, through its focus on individual needs, provides an exciting frontier for optimizing metabolism. By understanding how our unique biological makeup responds to different foods, we can harness the power of nutrition to create perfectly tailored diets. This expands the potential to enhance overall health, unlock energy, and hit those fitness goals.

However, it's important to remember that while your diet can greatly influence your metabolism, so can lifestyle factors, such as physical activity level, sleep duration and quality, and stress levels. Balancing all these components combined with a precision nutrition approach can truly maximize your metabolic potential, leading to sustainable health and well-being.

To conclude, embarking on a journey to boost your metabolism is not a short-term commitment to a fad diet. It's about understanding and making peace with your body's unique metabolic needs, finding joy in nourishing it with precisely what it needs, and reaping the rewards in the form of energy and health. Remember, your metabolism is not your enemy; it's a crucial part of you that just needs the right fuel to function optimally. As we continue to discover more about the intricate relationships between nutrition, metabolism, and health, the power of precision nutrition becomes more evident. By arming ourselves with this knowledge, we can make more empowered, personalized, and effective nutrition decisions for a healthier, more energetic life.

Chapter 4. Debunking Metabolic Myths: Fact vs Fallacy

Just as urban legends pervade popular culture, so too have a number of misconceptions spread through the wellness world, often muddying public understanding about metabolism. In this section, we aim to clarify the facts from fiction and offer you a trusted source for information. Armed with accurate knowledge, you can develop an effective strategy for boosting metabolic function and achieving your health goals.

4.1. Understanding Metabolism

Before diving into the myths, it's important to have a solid foundation of what metabolism actually is. Simply put, metabolism is all the chemical processes that happen in your body to keep you alive and functioning. These processes ultimately control your body's energy use and enable the growth and repair of cells. These vital processes need a careful balance - they can speed up (accelerate) or slow down (decelerate) depending on a range of factors such as age, sex, physical activity, hormonal balance, and even the type of foods we eat.

4.2. Myth 1: Skinny People Have Faster Metabolisms

This common myth likely stems from observations of individuals who seem to eat whatever they want without gaining weight. However, research indicates that larger bodies actually require more energy and therefore burn more calories—even at rest. A study published in the American Journal of Clinical Nutrition found that obese subjects had significantly higher resting metabolic rates than their lean counterparts. This dispels the widespread assumption that overweight individuals have slower metabolism.

4.3. Myth 2: Metabolism Cannot be Controlled

Though genetics do influence our metabolism, implying that it can't be controlled is a fallacy. It's true that you can't alter your age, sex, or height (all of which affect your metabolic rate), there are many factors within your control. Things like muscle mass, physical activity, and diet composition can drastically affect your metabolic rate.

For instance, regular exercise, especially strength training, can increase muscle mass and boost metabolism. Diet also play a pivotal role: foods rich in protein have been shown to increase metabolic rate more than other macronutrients due to the thermic effect of food (TEF), which refers to the energy required for digestion, absorption, and disposal of ingested nutrients.

4.4. Myth 3: You Gain Weight as you Age Because your Metabolism Slows Down

While metabolism does decrease with age, a shift linked to a loss of muscle mass and an increase in fat mass, this doesn't mean that weight gain is inevitable. Maintenance of muscle mass and engagement in regular physical activity can offset the decline in metabolic rate, helping to maintain a healthy weight as you age.

4.5. Myth 4: Eating Small, Frequent Meals Will Boost Your Metabolism

Many believe that consuming small, frequent meals throughout the day will keep the metabolism revved up and facilitate weight loss. However, studies show no significant difference in weight loss between those consuming an equal number of calories spread throughout the day versus concentrated in fewer meals. It's the total calories consumed versus those burned that matter most for weight control.

4.6. Myth 5: All Calories Are Created Equal

While it's true that a calorie is a measure of energy, how different foods influence your metabolism can vary drastically. As mentioned, protein-rich foods increase metabolism more than carbohydrates or fats due to TEF. Plus, fiber-rich whole foods can help you feel full longer, helping to reduce calorie intake. Moreover, processed and sugary foods can lead to inflammation and insulin resistance, negatively impacting your metabolism.

This chapter has highlighted the most common myths about metabolism, guided you through the reality behind each misconception, and provided you with practical and science-backed knowledge to understand and optimize your metabolic rate. Remember: every little change can be a step toward better health and wellness. However, sustainable improvement requires patience and persistence more than quick fixes or magic formulas. As you continue your wellness journey, let this be your guiding principle.

Chapter 5. Cracking the Code of Macronutrients

Understanding macronutrients – proteins, carbohydrates, and fats – is pivotal to managing your metabolic rate; these primary sources of energy play distinct roles in fueling your body. By decoding their functions, you can make informed dietary decisions for optimal health and wellbeing.

5.1. Protein: The Building Blocks of Life

The word 'protein' is derived from the Greek word 'proteios', meaning 'primary'. Indeed, protein has an indispensable role in the body – from growth and repair, to immune function and creating metabolic reactions. Amino acids, known as the 'building blocks' of proteins, are essential for creating enzymes, antibodies, hormones, and new tissue cells. Protein also assists in preserving lean muscle mass, which is vital for a robust metabolism.

Your body cannot store protein, so regular intake through diet is essential. The recommended dietary intake for an average adult is 0.8 grams per kilogram of body weight. If you're physically active, you may need more. Good sources include lean meats, poultry, fish, eggs, dairy products, legumes, nuts and seeds.

5.2. Carbohydrates: Your Body's Premium Fuel

Carbohydrates, derived from plant-based foods, are your body's main energy source. They provide immediate fuel for your cells, particularly brain cells. Carbohydrates can be divided into three categories: sugars (simple carbohydrates), starches (complex carbohydrates), and fiber.

Sugar provides instant energy and is found in fruits, vegetables and dairy products. Starches, found in foods like potatoes and grains, offer sustained energy by gradually releasing sugar into your bloodstream. Fiber promotes gut health and can be found in whole grains, legumes, and fruits.

While carbohydrates are essential, not all are created equal. Choose whole grains, fruits, vegetables, and legumes over processed carbohydrates.

The Dietary Guidelines for Americans recommends that carbohydrates make up 45 to 65 percent of your total daily calories. So, if you get 2,000 calories a day, between 900 and 1300 calories should be from carbohydrates. This translates to between 225 and 325 grams of carbohydrates a day.

5.3. Fats: Vital for Essential Functions

Contrary to common belief, fats are essential for optimum health. They assist in vitamin and mineral absorption, provide energy, create essential fatty acids that the body cannot produce, and are vital for hormonal production. Fats can be categorized into saturated, unsaturated, and trans fats.

While saturated and trans fats have been linked to health issues, unsaturated fats are beneficial. Monounsaturated fats and polyunsaturated fats, including omega-3 and omega-6 fatty acids, may decrease your risk of heart disease by improving related risk factors.

Good sources of healthy fats include olive oil, avocados, nuts, seeds, and cold-water fish like salmon and tuna. The Dietary Guidelines recommend that 20 to 35 percent of your daily calorie intake should come from fats.

5.4. Balancing Macronutrients: Key to Enhanced Metabolism

Understanding macronutrients lays the foundation for a balanced diet. Protein, carbohydrates, and fats each have unique roles and are mutually dependent. Following a diet that includes an ideal balance of proteins, carbohydrates, and fats can potentially increase satiety, maintain lean muscle mass, fuel your daily activities, and stabilize blood sugar levels.

Striking the right balance can be challenging. It's not a one-size-fits-all approach and individual requirements can vary. Factors such as age, sex, weight, height, level of physical activity, metabolic health, and personal goals (e.g., weight loss, muscle gain, maintaining health) can influence your macronutrient needs.

Meeting with a registered dietitian can provide a starting point to understand your individual needs, but exploration and trial-and-error is often the key to discovering what works best for your body. Establishing a well-rounded dietary strategy, filled with a variety of whole foods, is the cornerstone for maximizing your metabolism - and health.

Remember, the journey to optimizing your metabolism isn't a race, but rather a steady journey of discovery and commitment to your health. Start from where you are and make gradual tweaks to your diet, paying attention to how you feel along the way. Engage in regular physical activity. Stay hydrated. Rest well. And practice mindful eating. These elements, coupled with understanding and balancing your macronutrient intake, can transform your metabolic health - and life.

Chapter 6. Exercise to Maximize Metabolism: Best Practices

Your body is a finely tuned machine, relying on a mix of complex processes to maintain a semblance of order and functionality. Central to these processes is your metabolism, the chemical dance that converts food into energy and dictates how efficiently that energy is used. To nourish your metabolism, promoting its optimal functioning, you must grasp the art of balance: balance in nutrition, balance in rest, and critically, balance in exercise.

6.1. The Biology of Metabolism and Exercise

To begin, we must understand metabolism's inner workings. Metabolism is essentially a bonding of biochemistry and biophysics, comprising anabolic (building up) and catabolic (breaking down) reactions. Exercise, essentially, challenges your metabolism by increasing energy demand, sparking increased use of both your fat and glucose stores.

Exercise doesn't just burn calories during the activity, it also impacts the rate at which your body burns calories even when at rest, known as your Basal Metabolic Rate (BMR). The more muscle mass you have, the more calories your body needs to maintain that muscle, thus increasing your BMR.

6.2. The Significance of Muscle Mass

Resistance training is a powerful tool to boost your metabolism. It increases muscle mass and strengthens your body, fostering improved metabolic health. Research suggests that a pound of muscle burns approximately 7-10 calories a day, while a pound of fat burns only 2-3 calories.

Your muscle mass acts as a metabolic powerhouse in your body, and increasing it through strength training exercises can create a metabolic shift towards increased calorie-burning, thus fueling weight loss and enhanced fitness.

6.3. The Role of Cardiovascular Training

While strength training advances muscle mass, cardiovascular exercises also play a pivotal role in enhancing your metabolism. Cardio exercises like jogging, swimming, and cycling increase your heart rate, intensify calorie burning during the workout, and improve overall cardiovascular health.

High-intensity interval training (HIIT), a strategy that alternates short bouts of intense exercise with recovery periods, has shown to particularly elevate metabolic rates. HIIT workouts have been linked to increased fat oxidation, improved insulin sensitivity, and a post-exercise state called Excess Post-exercise Oxygen Consumption (EPOC), which enables your body to burn calories long after the workout has concluded.

6.4. Fusing Strength and Cardio: Synergy in Exercise

For optimal metabolic health, it is recommended to integrate both resistance and cardiovascular exercise into your routine. This not only dials up the metabolic benefits but also wards off monotony, keeping you motivated on your journey towards enhanced fitness.

To implement this, you could try circuit training, which includes short bouts of resistance exercises with little to no rest in between, effectively merging the benefits of strength and cardio exercises.

6.5. The Importance of Consistency and Progression

Whichever form of exercise you choose, remember that consistency is key. Do something that you love, so it becomes a part of your lifestyle rather than a chore. Progress over perfection should be your mantra.

Simultaneously, it's critical to challenge yourself. Gradually increase the intensity, duration, or frequency of your workouts to continue making metabolic gains. This concept, termed 'progressive overload', helps avoid workout plateaus and provides constant stimulation for muscle growth, fuelling your metabolic flame.

6.6. Rest, Recovery and Metabolism

Along with putting in hard work during the exercise, it is equally important to allow your body to rest and recover. Recovery refuels energy stores, repairs muscle tissue, and plays a vital role in the benefits realized from the workout.

Adequate sleep is one of the most effective recovery tools and is linked to key metabolic functions like glucose regulation and hormonal balance. Moreover, sleep deprivation can influence appetite regulation, leading to potential overeating and weight gain, further inhibiting metabolic efficiency.

6.7. A Fluid Relationship: Hydration and Metabolism

Hydration also has a substantial influence on metabolic health. Water is crucial for metabolizing stored fat and carbohydrates. Moreover, water-induced thermogenesis can increase your metabolic rate, promoting calorie burning. To keep your metabolic engine well-oiled, ensure you're hydrating adequately.

Exercise truly is a love letter to your metabolism. It stimulates muscle growth, burns calories, and incites processes that continue to burn calories long after the workout. But remember, there are no quick fixes. You need patience, persistence, and commitment.

Embrace a comprehensive approach to fitness – combining strength and cardiovascular exercise, prioritizing rest and recovery, and maintaining hydration and nutrition. Reclaim your metabolic power with fitness, empowering your body to be more efficient, strong, and robust. Your metabolism isn't a mystery; it's a puzzle, and exercise is a crucial piece of it. Only by fitting the pieces together can you see the full picture of metabolic health.

Chapter 7. Emotional Health's Impact on Metabolism

Frankly, there has long been a prevailing perception that the state of our metabolism is strictly tied to the physical aspects of our lives, with focus resting on diet and exercise. However, recent scientific research has revealed the deep-seated connection between our emotional health and metabolic wellness.

7.1. Understanding Emotions and Metabolism

Before we delve further into the relationship between emotional health and metabolism, it is imperative to understand the fundamental basics of both. Emotions are subjective, conscious experiences that evoke certain physiological responses. They are typically categorized into positive (e.g., happiness, love) and negative (e.g., sadness, anger).

On the other hand, metabolism refers to the set of chemical reactions that maintain our body's life processes. It includes anabolism (building up) and catabolism (breaking down) processes. These metabolic reactions lead to energy production, enabling bodily functions like growth, reproduction, response to the environment, and survival.

7.2. The Connection: Psychoneuroendocrinology

Psychoneuroendocrinology, the scientific field studying the

interaction between the endocrine system, nervous system, and psychological well-being, has shown the significant impact of stress and emotions on metabolic health. This interaction occurs mainly through the hypothalamic-pituitary-adrenal (HPA) axis, the body's central stress response system.

Chronic psychological stress activates the HPA axis, leading to the release of cortisol, commonly known as the stress hormone. Excessive cortisol interferes with the body's metabolic processes as it encourages the body to store fat around the abdomen, leading to weight gain and increased risk of metabolic disorders.

7.3. The Effect of Negative Emotions

Negative emotions such as stress, anxiety, and depression can inherently affect our eating behaviors and physical activity levels. Stress can incite overeating or under-eating, both of which significantly affect metabolic rate and overall metabolic health. Some people tend to soothe their emotional distress through "emotional eating", often opting for high-calorie comfort foods that adversely impact metabolism.

7.4. The Healing Power of Positive Emotions

Conversely, research demonstrates that positive emotions can fortify our metabolism. When we're in a state of joy, peace, or love, our body releases serotonin and oxytocin. These hormones not only make us feel good but also have a positive effect on our digestion, nutrient absorption, and overall metabolism. So it's not only what we eat but also how we feel when we eat that matters.

Moreover, happiness and contentment can motivate you to maintain a healthy exercise routine, which in turn enhances your metabolic function, contributing to overall physical health.

7.5. Balancing Emotions for Metabolic Health

It's clear that emotional health significantly contributes to metabolic wellbeing, but what practical steps can you take to nurture your emotional health? Begin by recognizing emotions and their triggers. Next, use various strategies like mindfulness, meditation, and physical activity to manage stress levels and promote positive emotional health.

A balanced diet, regular physical activity, and adequate sleep all contribute to emotional wellbeing. Also, cognitive behavioral therapy (CBT) can be a potent tool in managing emotions and reducing adverse metabolic effects from chronic stress or depression.

Emotional self-care is a crucial part of the puzzle in optimizing metabolic health, and this recognition calls for an empathetic, multi-dimensional approach to wellness. Remember, every effort counts, even if it's as simple as taking a few moments each day to tune into your feelings or indulge in a hobby that brings you joy and peace.

7.6. Conclusion

We are indeed a complex interplay of emotions and physicality. Our emotional health profoundly impacts our physical health, including our metabolism. Gaining awareness about this connection equips us with the knowledge to better manage our overall health. It's a holistic dance of physicality and emotions, and when we learn to choreograph this dance well, metabolic health invariably improves. So, embrace your feelings, understand them, and manage them effectively for metabolic wellbeing.

Let this understanding serve as a stepping stone in your journey towards achieving an optimal metabolic rate. Keep in mind that a well-balanced emotional state can lead to a healthier and happier life, featuring not only a better metabolic rate but also an enriched quality of life.

Welcome a robust metabolism by welcoming better emotional health. First, we accept; then, we prosper!

Chapter 8. Cultivating Healthy Habits for a Supercharged Metabolism

In the quest for a supercharged metabolism, cultivating healthy habits is an essential piece of the puzzle. This journey begins with unraveling the layers of nutritional knowledge, followed by understanding the necessary physical activity and finally, aligning the mind towards a healthier lifestyle.

8.1. Understanding Your Metabolic Necessities

Every individual carries unique metabolic needs, depending on various factors ranging from genetic predisposition to lifestyle design, body composition, and even sleep patterns. At the base of it all, however, are some universal nutritional necessities: a balanced meal, adequate hydration, and regular meal timings.

Balance is the key when it comes to your meal. Sufficient amounts of macro and micronutrients ensure that your body can carry out its functions optimally. Protein is generally hailed as the hero when it comes to metabolism. This is not just because protein-rich foods push your body to burn more calories during digestion (the thermic effect of food), but also because they aid in building lean muscle mass, which is metabolically more active than fat cells.

Including a broad spectrum of fruits and vegetables in your diet ensures an optimal intake of vitamins, minerals, and fibers. These not only help in keeping satiety levels high but also facilitate the smooth functioning of various metabolic processes. Regular consumption of fiber has also been linked to improved metabolic health, highlighting its significance in our diets.

Hydration, another critical factor, is much more than just quenching your thirst. Every metabolic process in your body, including calorie burning, needs water. Further, being dehydrated can slow down your metabolism and hence, negatively impact your weight loss efforts.

Lastly, your body loves routine. Regular meal timings can potentially improve metabolic health by positively influencing the body's circadian rhythms. These natural internal clocks play an influential role in regulating our metabolism.

8.2. The Role of Exercise in Metabolic Health

While nutrition is crucial for sustained metabolic health, there is no denying the role of physical activity. It's a thoughtful blend of cardio, strength training, and active rest that forms the base of a healthy metabolic rate.

Cardio, or cardiovascular exercises like brisk walking, jogging, swimming, biking, etc., not only burn considerable calories during the workout but also potentially enhance your metabolic rate for several hours after the exercise. This phenomenon is known as 'afterburn' or the excess post-exercise oxygen consumption (EPOC).

Strength training literally strengthens your metabolic health, by increasing your Resting Metabolic Rate (RMR). As your muscular strength and endurance grow, your body requires more energy (calories) to function even at rest. This form of exercise is particularly beneficial for long-term weight management.

'Active rest' refers to activities that help in recovery and relaxation of the body. These include practices like Yoga, Tai Chi, or even a leisurely walk. While these might not directly boost your metabolism, they contribute to overall health and wellness, thereby indirectly influencing metabolic health.

8.3. Mental Mettle: Mindset and Motivation

The adjustment to healthier habits is not just physical; it is psychological as well. Aligning your mind towards a new lifestyle requires sustained motivation, patience, and resilience.

Goal setting can be an extremely effective tool for this. A well-structured goal not only provides motivation but also keeps you on your path by providing a well-defined sense of direction. It's important, however, to prioritize practical and achievable goals over improbable ones to prevent self-defeat.

Your relationship with food also plays an important role in sustaining these healthier habits. Breaking away from the 'diet' mindset, viewing food as nourishment rather than numbers, appreciating the flavors, and truly savoring your meals can enhance the sustainability of these habits.

The role of stress is another factor that cannot be undermined. Chronic stress can affect both our eating behaviors as well as our metabolic health. Adopting regular stress-management practices like meditation, deep breathing, or hobbies is hence crucial for cultivating these healthier habits.

8.4. Sleep and Metabolic Health

Sleep potentially influences our metabolism and vice versa. The quality and quantity of sleep are important determinants of hunger hormones like Ghrelin (the 'hunger hormone') and Leptin (the 'satiety hormone'). These, in turn, impact our food intake and hence our metabolism.

Moreover, disrupted sleep or a lack of sleep has been linked to adverse metabolic conditions like obesity and type 2 diabetes. Incorporating a regular sleep schedule, adequate sleep hygiene practices, and prioritizing sleep quality and quantity, therefore, emerges as an integral part of this journey.

In conclusion, while the process is linear on paper, in reality, all these factors interact and intertwine with each other, determining the output - a supercharged metabolism. As you embark on this journey of transformation, remember to enjoy the process. After all, it is the small changes that weave the biggest transformations. As the adage goes, "The greatest wealth is health." Embrace these changes, preserve your health, and let your metabolism be your staunchest ally in this lifelong journey toward holistic health.

Chapter 9. Precision Fitness Techniques: Bringing Theory into Practice

The realm of fitness is no longer confined to merely sweating it out at the gym. it's about targeted, science-driven techniques designed to align with your unique bodily needs and optimize your metabolic functioning. While theory is vital for understanding the fundamental aspects, practice makes the magic happen.

9.1. Understanding Your Body

To begin with, it's essential to recognize that everybody is unique, with its specific metabolic rate, body composition, and varying physical capabilities. Therefore, it's critical to understand your body's particular needs before developing a precision fitness regime.

If possible, arrange for a comprehensive physical evaluation that includes muscle-to-fat ratio, resting metabolic rate tests, VO2 max (a measure of aerobic fitness), and flexibility tests. This evaluation will provide you with a detailed picture of your body's current fitness status and the areas that could use some improvement. Use these insights to tailor your fitness routine.

Integrating this personalized understanding with the Precision Fitness Techniques, we can bring the theory into practice and develop the best-suited fitness program for you.

9.2. Training Intensity and Energy Systems

Every activity we perform, from lifting weights to running or even day-to-day chores, uses energy. Our bodies operate on three primary energy systems: the ATP-PC system, the glycolytic system, and the oxidative system. Knowing which energy system your workout primarily uses can help you optimize your training intensity and get the most benefit from your training sessions.

For example, the ATP-PC system and the glycolytic system are predominantly used during high-intensity, short-duration workouts, such as weight lifting or sprinting. The oxidative system, however, is employed during low-intensity activities that last a longer duration like long-distance running.

9.3. High-Intensity Interval Training (HIIT)

High-Intensity Interval Training, or HIIT, is a modern fitness approach that alternates between short bursts of intense exercise followed by brief periods of rest or lower-intensity exercise. It is designed to burn a substantial amount of calories in less time while effectively improving cardiovascular and respiratory health.

Scientifically, HIIT stimulates a higher rate of metabolism post-workout - a phenomenon known as Excess Post-exercise Oxygen Consumption (EPOC), which means you continue to burn calories even after the workout is over. Start with 10-minute HIIT workouts and steadily increase your duration and intensity.

9.4. Resistance Training

Resistance training exercises are a cornerstone when it comes to boosting your metabolism. They increase muscle mass, and more muscles translate into more calories burned, even while at rest. By integrating weight training sessions into your fitness regimen, you can effectively enhance your Basal Metabolic Rate (BMR).

Remember, begin with lighter weights focusing on your form and then gradually increase the weight as your strength improves.

9.5. Rest, Recover, Repeat

Physical activities form just one-half of Precision Fitness Techniques; the remaining half is dedicated to effective resting strategies. It's during rest that the body repairs muscles, adapts to the exercise, and becomes stronger.

Ensure you get 7-9 hours of sleep every night. Rotate your workout routines to allow muscles the time to recover. Cross-training, alternatively focusing on different body parts in different sessions, is a smart way to prevent overuse of a particular muscle group.

Implementing these Precision Fitness Techniques will help you bring theory into practice. Remember that it's not about drastic changes but consistent efforts. Once you've established these techniques as part of your routine, you'll see a notable improvement in your metabolism, leading to a healthier, fit, and more energetic life.

Purchase this Special Report today, and watch yourself progress into the best version of yourself. Say goodbye to a one-size-fits-all approach, and welcome to the era of Precision Fitness Techniques, designed just for you!

Remember, the journey of a thousand miles begins with one step. Each step you take towards precision fitness is a step towards greater health, vitality, and an optimally functioning metabolism. The power is within you – it's time to unleash it!

Chapter 10. Meal Planning Tips to Boost Your Metabolism

A marked aspect in the paradigm shift towards achieving optimal metabolic health is the upturn and adoption of strategic meal planning. Benefiting from the fruits of methodology and intentionality in this sphere could signify the difference between average and exceptional metabolic health. Elevating metabolic health from a mere biological function into a higher realm of lifelong health and vitality begins at the dining table.

10.1. Understanding Your Metabolic Needs

The very first step before you build your nutrient-packed, metabolism-boosting meal plan, is to understand exactly what your body needs. An integral piece of the metabolic puzzle is to recognize that each person's dietary needs are unique and largely depend on age, gender, activity level, and underlying health issues.

Diana Austen, a leading nutritionist explains, "Because of the variations in our genetic makeup, daily routines, and overall health, the 'one-size-fits-all' approach doesn't apply to nutrition and metabolism". Hence, it's necessary to take into account personal variables, such as macronutrient requirements, calorie intake and food sensitivities, for a more exact and effective metabolic diet plan.

10.2. High-Protein Foods

A primary and essential element in meal planning to boost

metabolism is the inclusion of adequate protein. According to a study published in The American Journal of Clinical Nutrition, a high-protein diet can increase metabolism, reduce appetite, and stimulate weight loss.

Lean meats, eggs, dairy, legumes, seafood, and nuts are examples of protein-packed foods. It's important to ensure that each meal and snack contain a source of protein. This not only helps to keep hunger at bay and regulate blood sugar levels, but also aids in muscle recovery and growth post-exercise.

Sample meal: Grilled chicken breast with quinoa and steamed vegetables.

10.3. Fiber-Rich Foods

Fiber is another component you should aim to maximize in your meals for its metabolic benefits. These involve enhancing digestive health, reducing cholesterol levels, protecting against diseases, and aiding weight management. Consuming your fill of both soluble and insoluble fibers, from a variety of fruits, vegetables, and whole grains can significantly improve metabolic functions.

Sample meal: A large salad with mixed greens, tomatoes, cucumbers, carrots, boiled black beans, avocado, and a drizzle of balsamic vinaigrette.

10.4. Healthy Fats

While once vilified, fats have now taken center-stage in many health-conscious diet plans due to their metabolic properties. Healthy fats, such as polyunsaturated and monounsaturated fats found in avocados, nuts, seeds, fatty fish, and olive oil, can improve metabolic health, provide energy, and fuel weight loss. It's important to add these healthy fats to your diet, but in moderate amounts, as they're calorie dense.

Sample meal: Grilled salmon with avocado and wild rice.

10.5. Regular Hydration

Remember, water is a critical part of your metabolism-boosting meal plan. Adequate hydration is essential for every cellular function in the body, including metabolism. Aim for at least 8 glasses of water per day, and more if you're physically active.

10.6. Effective Meal Timing

Another point to take into account is meal timing, which surprisingly, plays a pivotal role in boosting metabolism. Frequent, small, balanced meals throughout the day can keep your metabolic furnace burning steadily. A good guideline is to aim for three main meals and two to three healthy snacks a day.

Sample snack: Greek yogurt with fresh mixed berries and a drizzle of honey.

10.7. Supplements to Consider

Certain natural supplements can complement your meal plan to further boost metabolism and overall health. Some of these include green tea extract, caffeine, and spices like black pepper and capsaicin. However, it is paramount to consult with your physician or a nutritionist before adding a supplement routine to your diet.

Taken together, these meal planning tips provide a solid foundation to create a personalized, powerful, and sustainable metabolism-boosting diet. Remember, it's not about a complete dietary overhaul overnight, but a progressive shift towards healthier eating habits and better metabolic health. So, go on and wield the power of meal planning to turn up your metabolic furnace and inspire your optimal health journey!

Chapter 11. The Future of Metabolic Health

Understanding the principles of metabolism and how to maximize its potential is more than a current wellness trend, it signals a shift into the future of metabolic health. Groundbreaking strides are consistently being made in the fields of exercise and nutritional science, bringing with it an exciting anticipation of what lays ahead. The focus of this chapter is to provide a forward-looking perspective on the subject, allowing each of us to see not just where we are now, but also where we could be in the future.

11.1. Unleashing the Power of Precision Nutrition

The concept of Precision Nutrition is not entirely novel, but the real-world implementation is becoming more streamlined and accessible today. This empowers us to make food choices that work best for our personal genetic makeup, gut microbiota, and lifestyle factors.

Scientific advances are improving our ability to analyze individual metabolic responses to various foods, and the roles of different bacteria in our gut flora. Terms that were once obscure – like our 'microbiome' – are now becoming more familiar. We are understanding more about how the thousands of different types of bacteria inside us interact with the food we eat, influencing our metabolic responses.

Biotech companies are developing personalized nutrition tests that can provide insights into our unique metabolic responses. In the future, these kinds of tailored dietary tools may become commonplace, making it easier for each of us to make the best decisions for our bodies.

11.2. Evolution of Exercise and Training Techniques

Similar to nutrition, exercise is not a one-size-fits-all solution. The future of metabolic health includes the rise of personalized training programs based on genetics, to ensure each workout optimally boosts our metabolic rate.

Current research is forging a path towards a deeper understanding of how genes impact our response to exercise. It's anticipated that one day soon we may be able to walk into a gym and receive a tailored exercise program based not only on our goals but also on our genetic makeup.

Moreover, emerging wearable technology provides real-time data about our workouts – heart rate, body temperature, lactic acid levels, and more — enabling precise measurements of the metabolic impact. As technology continues to evolve, these wearables could become instrumental in fine-tuning our exercise routines.

11.3. Metabolic Health and the Consciousness Evolution

Evolving cultural attitudes play a large role in the future of metabolic health. An increase in awareness and education has started shifting our focus from purely aesthetic goals to prioritizing health and longevity. It's about understanding that the metabolism is not simply a calorie-burning machine but an intricate system interconnected with every other part of our body.

This shift in consciousness allows us to view our body as a temple and the food we eat as fuel. Nutrition becomes a tool to nourish and strengthen our body, rather than a means to suppress our appetite. Similarly, exercise is appreciated as a form of movement that enhances our health, rather than a grueling task to burn off unwanted calories.

11.4. The Promise of Longevity Research

The future of metabolic health is invariably linked to longevity research. By understanding how metabolism affects aging, researchers are exploring ways to extend our healthspan – the number of years we stay healthy and active.

Recent studies reveal that various dietary and lifestyle interventions, such as intermittent fasting and regular exercise, can extend lifespan in various organisms, likely by impacting metabolic health. Several metabolic pathways — such as those involving insulin, mTOR, and sirtuins — are now recognized as key determinants of lifespan.

Further research might even open up the possibility of novel treatments that can slow aging by tweaking these metabolic pathways. It remains to be seen how these findings will translate into human life extension, but the future certainly looks promising.

11.5. Reclaiming Metabolic Health: A Return to Basics

As we look ahead, we may find that the future of metabolic health involves a return to some of the basic aspects of our ancestral lifestyles. Movements such as functional training and paleo nutrition have gained interest in recent years, showing a desire to return to more natural ways of eating and moving.

Embracing whole, nutrient-dense foods rather than processed ones, engaging in natural movement rather than isolated exercises, and prioritizing rest and recovery to support our metabolic health are all future trends to watch.

In conclusion, the future of metabolic wellness lies in blending the best of what modern science has to offer with a deep respect for our body's natural processes. It envisions a future where we can all take a proactive stance towards our health, enabling us to live not just longer, but also better. It's an exciting prognosis, full of promise and potential. As metabolic science advances, so does our ability to achieve and maintain optimal health. Indeed, the future of metabolic health holds great promise and potential, keeping us all on our toes as we watch it unfold.